Medical Medium Celery Juice Recipes: The Healing Power of Celery Juice

by Lara Smith

ISBN: 978-1-950171-51-4

Disclaimer:
The information provided in this book is designed to provide helpful information on the subjects discussed. The publisher and author are not responsible for any specific health or allergy needs that may require medical supervision and are not liable for any damages or negative consequences from any treatment, action, application or preparation, to any person reading or following the information in this book.

Table of Contents

Introduction

CELERY JUICE CAN HEAL YOU

When it comes to maintaining our health and living a healthy life, a lot of us still see it as a very expensive venture. But truth be told, it's not as luxurious as the society has termed it to be.

Ever heard of the miraculous vegetable "Celery"? Surprising many don't know about the highly beneficial attributes of the unpopular Celery because its' rarely spoken of talk less of its health benefits. Unlike many vegetables widely known, Experts say that Celery juice has outstanding healing properties as it contains vital minerals that help in the following;

1. **Lowers blood pressure.** Celery contains Magnesium, Phthalides, calcium, folate manganese and Potassium and high water content which can help those with high blood pressure.
2. **Great for thyroid recovery treatment**. Celery juice has helped many with thyroid disorders when taken daily. It helps in combating and cleansing the body of the Epstein-Barr virus, very common in the thyroid. Celery can also assist in boosting the production of key thyroid hormones.
3. **Serves as a natural detoxifier.** This doesn't mean we have to do away with green tea, and other detoxifying regimens. But we get bored with

routines sometimes and trying out a cup of celery juice will do you more good and it is also cheap.

4. **Reliefs to presence of inflammation**. Celery's anti-inflammatory property goes further to promote using Luteolin a powerful flavonoid that acts as an antioxidant thereby improving the well-being of the gut lining and helps to regulate successful digestion and the breaking down of food ingested for the whole day; thereby reducing digestive related challenges. Celery juice ingested daily will gradually repair and restore the stomach PH levels.

5. **Reduces the risk of heart disease.** Celery juice reduces the risk of stroke and anomalies in the arteries.
6. **Decreases the risk of liver disease** by aiding proper liver detoxification
7. **Celery Juice helps in guarding the body's nervous system**. Celery juices serve as a livewire that assists the body's nervous system and has the ability to calm the nervous system because of its blood purifying properties.
8. **Celery juice increases and fortifies your bile.** When the bile is strong it breaks down fats and eliminates waste from the body faster.

Asides from its anti-inflammatory properties, Celery is very rich in vitamin K, B6 and C and also a great source of Fiber.

PROPER WAYS TO TAKE CELERY JUICE

1. To be taken immediately after juicing or consumed in the space of 24 hours.
2. Celery juice is most effective when taken first thing in the morning and given 15 mins window before any meal.
3. Don't be startled at the loose stools; it will pass as your body repairs itself.
4. If you feel the Celery juice is bitter, add a cucumber or an apple instead of artificial additives or sweeteners in other not to destroy its fiber components and defeat the initial motive. Or more so, blend the whole celery in a smoothie.

5 Steps To Creating The Perfect Smoothie Experience

Step 1: If you are new to juicing, I recommend Starting out with these vegetables, as they are the easiest to Digest and tolerate:

1. Celery
2. Fennel
3. Cucumbers

These three aren't as nutrient dense as the dark green vegetables. Once you get used to the 3 vegetables listed above, you can start adding the more nutritionally valuable but less palatable vegetable into your juice.

Step 2: When you've acclimatized yourself to juicing, you can start adding these vegetables.

1. Red Leaf lettuce
2. Green leaf lettuce
3. Romaine lettuce
4. Endive
5. Spinach

Step 3: After you are used to this, then you move on to the next step

1. Cabbage
2. Chinese Cabbage
3. Bok Choy

An interesting Side note: Cabbage juice is one of the most healing nutrients for ulcer repair as it is a huge source of vitamin U.

Step 4: When you're ready, move on to adding herbs to your juicing. Herbs also makes wonderful combination, and here are two that works exceptionally well:

1. Parsley
2. Cilantro

Nb: You need to be cautious with cilantro, as many cannot tolerate it well. If you are new to juicing, you might probably want to hold off on cilantro. These are more challenging to consume but they are highly beneficial.

Step 5: Only use one or two of this leave as they are highly bitter:

1. Kale
2. Collard greens
3. Mustard greens
4. Boundelion greens

The Best way to store the juice is in a Glass mason jar with a lid and keep it in the Fridge

Let's Get Started

Celery Juice can be made by Rinsing the celery and running it through a juicer. Drink immediately for best results. Alternatively, you can chop the celery and blend it in a high-speed blender until smooth. Strain well and drink immediately For Best Result.

In this Book we have included a mix of celery with other powerful ingredients for Those who have preferences to help Restore health in people who suffer from a vast range of chronic and mystery illnesses and symptoms, among them eczema, addiction, ADHD, thyroid disorders, diabetes, fatigue, brain fog, acne, SIBO, disorders, Lyme disease, eating disorders, autoimmune and eye problems .

There are unlimited combinations, but I recommend not adding too many ingredients per smoothie. Simple is usually better. By experimenting with different combinations, you will be able to come up with something that you and your whole family will love.

These Delicious Celery Juice and smoothies will help you heal your gut and relieve digestive disorders amongst others.

Bananas Blast

Ingredients:

4 leaves kale
2 celery stalks
2 bananas (Fresh or Frozen)
1 cup of strawberries or blueberries or raspberries (Fresh or Frozen)
2 cups of water

How you make it:

1. Place the kale leaves and water into the blender and blend until the mixture is a juice-like consistency.
2. Stop the blender and add the remaining ingredients. Blend until creamy.

Yummy Berries Smoothies

Ingredients:

4 cups spinach
2 celery stalks
1/2 cup of raspberries(Fresh or Frozen)
1/2 cup of strawberries (Fresh or Frozen)
2 bananas
1 1/2 cup of water, or enough water to blend into desired consistency.

How you make it:

1. Place the Spinach and water into the blender and blend until the mixture is a juice-like consistency.
2. Stop the blender and add the remaining ingredients. Blend until creamy.

Watermelon Cleansing Smoothies

Ingredients:

2 cups cubed seedless watermelon
1 whole cucumber, peeled, seeded, and coarsely chopped
1 large handful chopped kale
3 tablespoons fresh lime juice
1/4 cup chopped fresh mint
1/4 cup chopped fresh basil
1 cup ice cubes

How you make it:

1. Place the watermelon and cucumber in a blender, and blend until creamy and smooth.
2. Add the remaining ingredients and process again.
3. Drink ice cold.

Green Smoothie aficionados

Ingredients:

1 cup water
¼ cup beet chopped
¼ cup carrot chopped small
Small amount ginger
½ avocado
1 cup mild greens (spinach, kale, choy, sweet potato leaves)
1 cup strong greens (rocket, watercress or mustard leaves)
¼ cup cilantro/coriander
1 cup parsley
Sea salt
2 tbsp. lime juice
1 cup ice and blend again

How you make it:

1. First, Place beet, carrot, water and small amount of ginger into blender and blend until mixture is a green juice-like consistency.
2. Stop blender and add avocado, greens with the other remaining ingredients and blend.
3. Add 1 cup of ice and blend again until creamy.

Tips

To green it up even more add a stalk of celery or a cup of broccoli
Add some cayenne pepper and cumin

Mango Soft-n-Yummy Smoothie

Ingredients:

2-4 cups leaves of green leaf lettuce
2 ripe mangoes, peeled and pit removed
2 apples
1 banana
2 cups of water

How you make it:

1. Place the green lettuce leaves and water into the blender and blend until the mixture is a juice-like consistency.
2. Stop the blender and add the remaining ingredients. Blend until creamy.

Heveanly Dews Smoothie

Ingredients:

1/2 pear
1 cup chopped and seeded cucumber
1/4 cup chopped fresh dill
1 small avocado
1 cup baby spinach
2 tablespoons lime juice
1-inch knob fresh gingerroot, peeled
1 cup frozen pineapple
11/4 cups water
3 to 4 ice cubes

How you make it:

1. Place all the ingredients except the ice in a blender, and blend until smooth and creamy.
2. Add the ice and process again. Drink chilled.

Ultimate Cleansing Smoothies

Ingredients:

2 cups collard greens
2 celery stalks
1 cucumber
2 pears
1/2 inch ginger
1 lemon
1 cup water

How you make it:

1. Place the collard and water into blender and blend until mixture is a green juice-like consistency.
2. Stop blender and add the other remaining ingredients and blend.
3. Add ice if desired and blend again until creamy.

Peachy Dream Smoothie

This creamy dreamy treat is so tasty it can even be eaten as "ice cream"; simply transfer the smoothie into 4 small ramekins and freeze for about 10 minutes.

Ingredients:

1/2 avocado
1 cup frozen organic frozen peaches
1 frozen banana, cut into pieces
2 tablespoons fresh lemon juice
11/4 cups water
Handful of kale
3 to 4 ice cubes
Optional: 2 to 3 pitted dates

How you make it:

1. Place all the ingredients except the ice in a Blender, and blend until smooth and creamy.
2. Add the ice and dates (if using) and process again. Drink chilled.

Berry Bang

Ingredients:

1 cup water
1 cup raspberries (fresh or frozen)
1 cup other berries (fresh or frozen)
2 bananas
2 cups spinach (or mild greens in any combination)
Sea salt, cinnamon and vanilla

How you make it:

1. Place Spinach and water into blender and blend until mixture is a green juice-like consistency.
2. Stop blender and add remaining ingredients.
3. Blend until creamy.
4. Add ice and water for desired temperature and consistency

Fresh Spinach Smoothies

Ingredients:

1 cup water
2 cups pineapple (fresh or frozen)
1 avocado
1 cup mint leaves
1 cup of spinach leaves or other mild green

How To Make It:

Blend until Smooth then Add Ice and extra water to get to your desired temperature and consistency.

Salad Smoothie

First blend

1 cup water
¼ cup beet chopped
¼ cup carrot chopped small
Small amount ginger

Then add
½ avocado
1 cup mild greens (spinach, kale, choy, sweet potato leaves)
1 cup strong greens (rocket, watercress or mustard leaves)
¼ cup cilantro/coriander
1 cup parsley
Sea salt
2 tbsp lime juice
1 cup ice and blend again

Blend until mixture is a green juice-like consistency.
Serve Chilled

Juicy Dilly Dally

Ingredients:

1 cup kale
1 cup water
¼ cup dill
1 tomato
1 tbsp. lime juice
1 cup bok or pak choy (don't feel constrained. If you don't have kale and choy, just use 2 cups mild greens. Remember to vary your green intake)
½ avocado
OPTIONAL: 1 1/2 cups pineapple

How you make it:

5. Place kale, choy and water into blender and blend until mixture is a green juice-like consistency.
6. Stop blender and add remaining ingredients.
7. Blend until creamy.
8. Add ice and water for desired temperature and consistency

Delicious Dandelion Smoothie

Ingredients:

1/2 bunch red dandelion
1/2 small watermelon
1/2 cup strawberries
1 cup of grapes
1 cup water

How you make it:

1. Place the red dandelion and water into the blender and blend until the mixture is a juice-like consistency.
2. Stop the blender and add the remaining ingredients. Blend until creamy.

Ultimate Green Smoothies

Ingredients:

1 small bunch green kale
1 pint strawberries
3 small peaches
2 cups water

How you make it:

1. Place the green kale and water into the blender and blend until the mixture is a juice-like consistency.
2. Stop the blender and add the remaining ingredients. Blend until creamy.

Cabbage Cadillac

Ingredients:

1 cup spinach
1 cup cabbage
1 celery
1 cup almond milk
2 packets of stevia
1 cup of ice

How you make it:

1. Place all the ingredients into blender and blend until mixture is a green juice-like consistency.
2. Add the cup of ice and blend again until creamy.

Morning Dews Smoothies

Ingredients:

4 cups of kale
½ bunch of mint
4 ripe pears (Fresh or Frozen)
2 cups water

How you make it:

1. Place the kale and water into the blender and blend until the mixture is a juice-like consistency.
2. Stop the blender and add the remaining ingredients. Blend until creamy.

Healthy Body Smoothie

Ingredients:

Handful of almonds
1 cup water
2 dates
1 tsp vanilla essence
2 kiwi
¼ tsp salt
1 cup kale (or mild greens)
½ cup broccoli
Handful of sprouts

How you make it:

1. First, Place the almonds and water into blender and blend until mixture is a green juice-like consistency.
2. Stop blender and add dates, vanilla essence, greens with the other remaining ingredients and blend.
3. Add ice if desired and blend again until creamy.

Berry Bath

Ingredients:

1 cup water
1 cup raspberries (Fresh or frozen)
1 apple (minus the stalk, chopped)
¼ cup cilantro/coriander
1 celery stalk
1 1/2 cup mild greens
1 cup of Ice

How you make it:

1. Place all the ingredients into blender and blend until mixture is a green juice-like consistency.
2. Add ice and blend again until creamy.

Blue d'Bomb

Ingredients:

1/4 cups blueberries (Fresh or Frozen)
1/4 cups blackberries (Fresh or Frozen)
1 banana (Fresh or Frozen)
1/2 cups apple juice
1/3 cups raspberry sorbet

How you make it:

1. Put all ingredients into blender.
2. Blend until smoothie consistency is reached!

Apples Appealin'

Ingredients:

4 cups of kale
4 apples (Fresh or frozen)
½ lemon juice
1 cup ice

How you make it:

1. First, Place the kale and water into blender and blend until mixture is a green juice-like consistency.
2. Stop blender and add the other remaining ingredients and blend.
3. Add ice if desired and blend again until creamy.

Green Detoxifier

Ingredients:

1/2 head of lettuce
1 cup dandelion greens
2 celery sticks
2 apples
1 banana
1 cup of ice

How you make it:

1. First, Place the lettuce head and water into blender and blend until mixture is a green juice-like consistency.
2. Stop blender and add the other remaining ingredients and blend.
3. Add ice if desired and blend again until creamy.

Romaine Relish

Ingredients:

½ bunch Romaine
2 cups strawberries (Fresh or Frozen)
2 bananas (Fresh or Frozen)
2 cups water

How you make it:

Place the Romaine and water into the blender and blend until the mixture is a juice-like consistency.

Stop the blender and add the remaining ingredients. Blend until creamy.

Lemonade Loungin'

Ingredients:

1 small bunch dandelion greens (or substitute with spinach)
1 lemon (peeled)
2 large apples (Fresh or Frozen)
1 banana (Fresh or Frozen)
2 cups water

How you make it:

Place the dandelion greens and water into the blender and blend until the mixture is a juice-like consistency.

Stop the blender and add the remaining ingredients. Blend until creamy.

Apple n Blueberries Smoothie

Ingredients:

1 cup water
1 cup blueberries (frozen)
1 apple (without the stalk, chopped)
¼ cup dill
1 celery stalk
1 1/2 cups mild greens
Ice

How you make it:

1. Place all the ingredients into blender and blend until mixture is a green juice-like consistency.
2. Add ice and blend again until creamy.

Orange Oriental

Ingredients:

1/2 head romaine
2 stalks of celery
1 cup papaya
1 orange (Fresh or Frozen)
1 cup of red grapes (Fresh or Frozen)
2 cups water

How you make it:

1. Place the romaine head and water into the blender and blend until the mixture is a juice-like consistency.
2. Stop the blender and add the remaining ingredients.
3. Blend until creamy.

Mango Island Smoothie

Ingredients:

2-4 cups leaves of green leaf lettuce
2 ripe mangoes, peeled and pit removed
1 banana (Fresh or Frozen)
2 apples (Fresh or Frozen)
2 cups of water

How you make it:

1. First, Place the lettuce leaf and water into blender and blend until mixture is a green juice-like consistency.
2. Stop blender and add the other remaining ingredients and blend.
3. Add ice if desired and blend again until creamy.

Cucumber Cleansing

Ingredients:

2 cups collard greens
2 celery stalks
1 cucumber
2 pears
1/2 inch ginger
1 lemon
1 cup water

How you make it:

1. Place the collard greens and water into the blender and blend until the mixture is a juice-like consistency.
2. Stop the blender and add the remaining ingredients.
3. Blend until creamy.

Strawberry Sunrise

Ingredients:

1 cup water
1 cup strawberries (frozen or fresh)
2 kiwi
¼ cup dill
2 cups of mild greens (try bok choy, spinach or chickweed)
1 stalk celery
Ice

How you make it:

1. Place all the ingredients into blender and blend until mixture is a green juice-like consistency.
2. Add ice and blend again until creamy.

Dandelion Dews

Ingredients:

1/2 head of lettuce
1 cup dandelion greens
2 celery sticks
2 apples
1 banana

How you make it:

1. Place the lettuce head and water into the blender and blend until the mixture is a juice-like consistency.

2. Stop the blender and add the remaining ingredients.

3. Blend until creamy.

Slimin' Smoothies

Ingredients:

1/2 head romaine lettuce
2 stalks of celery
1 orange (Fresh or Frozen)
1 bunch red grapes (Fresh or Frozen)
1 cup water

How you make it:

1. Place the romaine lettuce head and water into the blender and blend until the mixture is a juice-like consistency.
2. Stop the blender and add the remaining ingredients.
3. Blend until creamy.

Brussels Bat

Ingredients:

12 Brussels sprouts
1 yellow grapefruit, peeled
2 cups mixed berries, frozen
2 bananas, frozen
1 apple
1 cup any type cooked whole grain or white bean
Stevia or agave to taste (optional)
3 cups water/ice

How you make it:

1. First, Place the Brussel sprout and ice into blender and blend until mixture is a green juice-like consistency.
2. Stop blender and add celery, orange, the red grapes and blend.
3. Add ice if desired and blend again until creamy.

Avocados Pudding Smoothie

Ingredients:

1 cup water
½ cup cashews (soaked if you have them available, dry will do)
3 dates (no stone. Or other dried fruit)
2 tbsp. carob
1 small avocado, or ½ large
2 cups mild greens
¼ - ½ tsp cinnamon
Vanilla
Pinch sea salt
1 cup ice or as needed

How you make it:

1. First, Place the cashews, dates and water into blender and blend until mixture is a green juice-like consistency.
2. Stop blender and add carob, green with the other remaining ingredients and blend.
3. Add 1 cup of ice and blend again until creamy.

Mango Smooth

Ingredients:

1 small pineapple (Fresh or Frozen)
1 large mango (Fresh or Frozen)
1 small head romaine
A piece of ginger
1 cup of ice

How you make it:

1. First, Place the lettuce and water into blender and blend until mixture is a green juice-like consistency.
2. Stop blender and add the other remaining ingredients and blend.
3. Add ice if desired and blend again until creamy.

Pear Refresher

Lots of green stuff, tons of flavor. Fennel definitely makes this a taste sensation. The salt gives it a flavor boost. Try it.

Ingredients:

1 stalk celery
1 pear
½ cup fennel
1 cup parsley
1 cup greens of your choice
1-2 tbsp. lemon optional
1 cup water
Pinch sea salt
Add ½ cup ice

How you make it:

1. Place all the ingredients into blender and blend until mixture is a green juice-like consistency.
2. Add ice and blend again until creamy.

Perfect Energizer

This Smoothie as it's called is gushing with vitamin C, this energizing drink is the perfect alternative to your morning break!

Ingredients:

1 orange, peeled and chopped (Fresh or Frozen)
1 kiwi, peeled and chopped
5 pitted dates
1/2 cup frozen pineapple
2 tablespoons hemp seeds
1/2 cup water
3 to 4 ice cubes

How you make it:

1. Place all the ingredients except the ice in a blender, and blend until smooth and creamy.
2. Add the ice and process again.
3. Drink chilled.

Conclusion

I want to encourage you to take this challenge today, to commit to something because when you commit to something and you actually do it and stick with it, it builds up the habit and the real power. When was the last time you had a goal you actually set Up and feel good about it, I want you to get this in your mind that we always need New Goals.

The healing attributes of Celery juice are infinite. It is important we take advantage of its healing power as it plays a fundamental role in the gut which is connected to our entire being.

Celery Juice has helped transformed lives, with lots of great testimonies. A glass of celery juice a day will keep the doctor away. Take Massive action in your life today, because your transformation would affect positive changes on you and everyone around you.

Thank You

If you follow religiously to The Medical Medium Celery Juice by Anthony Williams And some of the Smoothie recipes outlined in this book. You are going to be seeing great results in your body and health in just 10 days, because it is proven to work.

If you enjoyed the recipes in this book, please take the time to share your thoughts and post a positive review on Amazon, it would encourage me and make me serve you better. It'd be greatly appreciated!

CPSIA information can be obtained
at www.ICGtesting.com
Printed in the USA
LVHW012321020419
612783LV00007B/160/P